"Depression: A Roller Coaster Ride"

Swatantra Bahadur

Published by Swatantra Bahadur, 2023.

Disclaimer

The information presented in this book is intended for general informational purposes only and should not be relied upon as a substitute for professional advice or judgment. The author and publisher are not responsible for any action taken by readers based on the information provided in this book. Readers should seek appropriate professional advice or conduct their own research before making decisions related to the topics discussed in this book. The views expressed in this book are those of the author and do not necessarily reflect the views of the publisher.

"Depression: A Roller Coaster Ride"

Contents

I. Introduction

Depression is a common and serious mental health condition that affects millions of people worldwide. It is a mood disorder characterized by persistent feelings of sadness, hopelessness, and worthlessness. Depression can impact a person's thoughts, emotions, and behaviors, making it difficult for them to function in their daily lives. It is important to understand the symptoms, causes, and treatment options for depression to help individuals affected by this condition to manage their symptoms and lead fulfilling lives. In this outline, we will explore the different aspects of depression, including its symptoms, causes, types, diagnosis, treatment, and prevention.

1. Definition of depression

Depression is a mental health disorder characterized by persistent feelings of sadness, hopelessness, and loss of interest in activities that were once enjoyable. It is a mood disorder that affects a person's thoughts, feelings, and behaviors, leading to a variety of physical and emotional symptoms. Depression can be a serious condition that can affect a person's ability to function in their daily life, impacting their work, relationships, and overall quality of life. It is a common mental health issue, with millions of people worldwide experiencing some form of depression at some point in their lives.

· · · ·

2. DEPRESSION AND ANXIETY: What's the connection?

Depression and anxiety are two different mental health conditions, but they often coexist and can have a complex relationship. While they have some similar symptoms, such as feelings of worry and fear, they also have some important differences.

Depression is characterized by feelings of sadness, hopelessness, and loss of interest or pleasure in activities. Anxiety, on the other hand, involves excessive worry and fear about everyday situations or events, and can lead to physical symptoms such as sweating and rapid heartbeat.

The relationship between depression and anxiety can be cyclical. For example, someone with depression may experience anxiety as a symptom of their depression, while someone with anxiety may develop depression as a result of their constant worrying and fear.

Additionally, some people with anxiety may avoid certain situations or activities due to their fear, which can lead to feelings of sadness and isolation and eventually develop into depression.

It is important to note that depression and anxiety are treatable conditions, and a mental health professional can help develop a personalized treatment plan that addresses both conditions if they coexist.

3. Explanation of the prevalence of depression and anxiety and how they often coexist

Depression and anxiety are two of the most common mental health disorders, and they often coexist. According to the World Health Organization (WHO), depression is the leading cause of disability worldwide, affecting over 264 million people, and anxiety disorders affect over 284 million people globally.

The prevalence of depression and anxiety has increased in recent years, with factors such as stress, trauma, and changes in lifestyle contributing to the rise. Additionally, stigma surrounding mental health has decreased, leading more people to seek help and receive a diagnosis.

Depression and anxiety commonly coexist, with research suggesting that up to 50% of people diagnosed with depression also experience symptoms of anxiety, and vice versa. This comorbidity can make diagnosis and treatment more complex, as symptoms can overlap and require a personalized approach.

The coexistence of depression and anxiety can also have a significant impact on an individual's overall functioning, leading to difficulties in daily life, work, and relationships. This makes it essential to understand the connection between depression and anxiety and develop effective strategies for managing both conditions.

4. Depression in children and adolescents

Depression in children and adolescents is a serious mental health condition characterized by persistent feelings of sadness, hopelessness, and/or irritability. Children and adolescents with depression may also experience a range of physical symptoms, such as headaches, stomach aches, or changes in appetite or sleep patterns.

Depression in children and adolescents can affect their mood, behavior, and overall functioning, and can interfere with their ability to engage in daily activities, such as school, socializing, or hobbies. Depression in children and adolescents can also have a negative impact on their academic performance, relationships with peers and family members, and overall quality of life.

Some common symptoms of depression in children and adolescents may include:

1. Persistent feelings of sadness or hopelessness
2. Loss of interest in activities they used to enjoy
3. Irritability or anger
4. Low self-esteem or feelings of worthlessness
5. Changes in appetite or weight
6. Changes in sleep patterns
7. Fatigue or lack of energy
8. Difficulty concentrating or making decisions
9. Physical symptoms, such as headaches or stomach aches
10. Thoughts of death or suicide

Depression in children and adolescents can be caused by a range of factors, including genetics, brain chemistry, life stressors, and environmental factors. It is important for parents and caregivers to be aware of the symptoms of depression in children and adolescents and seek professional help if they suspect their child may be experiencing depression. With proper diagnosis and treatment, depression in children and adolescents can be effectively managed and treated.

2. Importance of understanding depression

Understanding depression is crucial because it is a widespread mental health condition that can have a significant impact on an individual's life. Depression can affect a person's ability to work, socialize, and enjoy their daily activities, leading to a lower quality of life. Additionally, depression is a leading cause of disability worldwide, with severe cases often requiring hospitalization or treatment in specialized mental health facilities.

Understanding depression can also help individuals identify the signs and symptoms of the condition in themselves or others. Early recognition and intervention of depression can improve the chances of successful treatment and reduce the risk of complications or worsening of the condition.

Lastly, destigmatizing depression and promoting awareness can encourage individuals to seek help for their mental health, reduce shame and fear associated with the condition, and improve overall mental health outcomes.

II. Understanding Depression in Children and Adolescents

Depression in children and adolescents is a serious mental health concern that affects a significant portion of the youth population. It is important to understand the signs, symptoms, and risk factors of depression in this age group in order to provide appropriate support and treatment.

Depression in children and adolescents can manifest in different ways than it does in adults. Children and adolescents may display irritability, behavioral problems, or physical complaints rather than the typical symptoms of sadness and hopelessness. It is important to recognize these alternative symptoms as signs of depression and seek appropriate treatment.

Risk factors for depression in children and adolescents include genetic factors, family history of depression or other mental health concerns, adverse childhood experiences, social isolation, and academic or social pressures. Early identification and intervention can help prevent the worsening of symptoms and the development of more severe mental health concerns.

Treatment for depression in children and adolescents often involves a combination of psychotherapy and medication. Cognitive-behavioral therapy (CBT) is a commonly used form of therapy that focuses on identifying negative thought patterns and developing coping skills. Medication, such as selective serotonin reuptake inhibitors (SSRIs), can be effective in treating depression in some cases.

Preventing depression in children and adolescents involves promoting healthy lifestyles, building resilience, and addressing risk factors. Early intervention and support from parents, caregivers, and mental health professionals can also help prevent the development of depression.

It is important to take depression in children and adolescents seriously and provide appropriate support and treatment. With the right care and support, children and adolescents with depression can recover and lead fulfilling lives.

1. Definition and symptoms of depression in children and adolescents

Depression in children and adolescents is a mental health condition characterized by persistent feelings of sadness, hopelessness, and a loss of interest in activities they once enjoyed. Depression in this age group may also be accompanied by physical symptoms, behavioral problems, or irritability.

Symptoms of depression in children and adolescents can vary, and may include:

1. Persistent sadness or hopelessness
2. Loss of interest or pleasure in activities once enjoyed
3. Changes in appetite or weight
4. Sleep disturbances, such as difficulty falling or staying asleep, or sleeping too much
5. Fatigue or loss of energy
6. Feelings of worthlessness or guilt
7. Difficulty concentrating or making decisions
8. Physical complaints such as headaches or stomach aches
9. Irritability or anger
10. Withdrawal from social activities or relationships

Children and adolescents with depression may also have thoughts of suicide or self-harm, which should be taken seriously and immediately addressed by a mental health professional.

It is important to note that these symptoms may also be present in other mental health conditions, such as anxiety or trauma-related disorders, and a thorough evaluation by a mental health professional is necessary to determine an accurate diagnosis.

2. Risk factors and causes of depression in children and adolescents

There are several risk factors and causes that can contribute to the development of depression in children and adolescents. Some of these include:

1. **Genetics:** Children and adolescents with a family history of depression or other mental health concerns may be at a higher risk for developing depression themselves.
2. **Adverse childhood experiences:** Traumatic events such as abuse, neglect, or exposure to violence can increase the risk of depression in children and adolescents.
3. **Social isolation:** Children and adolescents who feel socially isolated or have a difficult time making friends may be at a higher risk of

developing depression.

4. **Academic or social pressures:** The pressure to perform well in school, participate in extracurricular activities, or meet other expectations can contribute to stress and increase the risk of depression.

5. **Medical conditions:** Children and adolescents with chronic medical conditions or illnesses may be at a higher risk of developing depression.

6. **Substance use:** Substance use or abuse can increase the risk of depression in children and adolescents.

It is important to note that depression can be caused by a combination of these factors, and the exact cause of depression may be different for each individual. Identifying and addressing risk factors can help prevent the development of depression in children and adolescents. Early intervention and support from mental health professionals can also be beneficial in preventing the worsening of symptoms and the development of more severe mental health concerns.

3. Diagnosis and assessment of depression in children and adolescents

Diagnosing and assessing depression in children and adolescents involves a comprehensive evaluation by a mental health professional, such as a child and adolescent psychiatrist or clinical psychologist. The assessment may involve the following:

1. **Clinical interview:** The mental health professional may conduct a clinical interview with the child or adolescent, as well as their parents or caregivers, to gather information about symptoms, medical history, family history, and any other relevant information.

2. **Self-report measures:** The mental health professional may use self-report measures, such as questionnaires or surveys, to gather information about the child or adolescent's symptoms and experiences.

3. **Behavioral observations:** The mental health professional may observe the child or adolescent's behavior, mood, and social interactions in different settings, such as at home or school.

4. **Diagnostic criteria:** The mental health professional will use diagnostic criteria from the Diagnostic and Statistical Manual of Mental

Disorders (DSM-5) to determine if the child or adolescent meets the criteria for a diagnosis of depression.

It is important to note that depression in children and adolescents can present differently than in adults, and may involve more physical symptoms, such as headaches or stomach aches, rather than feelings of sadness or hopelessness. Additionally, it is common for children and adolescents to have co-occurring mental health conditions, such as anxiety or attention-deficit/hyperactivity disorder (ADHD), which may complicate the diagnosis and treatment of depression. A thorough assessment by a mental health professional is crucial for accurate diagnosis and appropriate treatment planning.

4. Differences between depression in children/adolescents and adults

Depression in children and adolescents can differ from depression in adults in several ways. Some of the key differences include:

1. **Symptoms:** Children and adolescents may experience different symptoms of depression than adults. For example, instead of feeling sad or hopeless, they may be irritable, angry, or have frequent temper tantrums. Physical symptoms such as headaches or stomach aches may also be more common in children and adolescents.

2. **Co-occurring conditions:** Children and adolescents with depression are more likely to have co-occurring mental health conditions, such as anxiety or ADHD, than adults with depression. This can complicate the diagnosis and treatment of depression in children and adolescents.

3. **Triggers:** Depression in children and adolescents may be triggered by different factors than depression in adults. For example, academic or social pressures may contribute to depression in children and adolescents, whereas work-related stress may contribute to depression in adults.

4. **Treatment:** The treatment of depression in children and adolescents may differ from the treatment of depression in adults. For example, psychotherapy, such as cognitive-behavioral therapy (CBT), may be the first-line treatment for children and adolescents with mild to moderate depression, whereas medication may be the first-line

treatment for adults with moderate to severe depression.

5. **Prognosis:** Depression in children and adolescents may have different long-term outcomes than depression in adults. For example, depression in children and adolescents may be more likely to recur and lead to a more chronic course of illness than depression in adults.

Understanding these differences is important for accurate diagnosis and appropriate treatment of depression in children and adolescents.

III. Impact of Depression on Children and Adolescents

Depression can have a significant impact on the lives of children and adolescents. It can affect their mood, behavior, and overall functioning, and can interfere with their ability to engage in daily activities, such as school, socializing, or hobbies.

Some of the ways in which depression can impact children and adolescents include:

1. **Academic performance:** Depression can affect a child's or adolescent's ability to concentrate and perform well in school. They may have difficulty completing assignments or may miss school due to fatigue or other physical symptoms.
2. **Relationships with peers and family members:** Children and adolescents with depression may withdraw from social activities and have difficulty making and maintaining friendships. They may also have conflict with family members, particularly if their depression leads to irritability or anger.
3. **Physical health:** Depression can have physical effects, such as changes in appetite, sleep patterns, and energy levels. Children and adolescents with depression may also be at higher risk for other health problems, such as obesity, heart disease, and substance abuse.
4. **Emotional well-being:** Depression can lead to persistent feelings of sadness, hopelessness, and worthlessness. Children and adolescents may also experience thoughts of death or suicide, which can be very distressing and require immediate attention.
5. **Risk-taking behaviors:** Some children and adolescents with depression may engage in risky behaviors, such as drug or alcohol use, reckless driving, or self-harm, as a way of coping with their symptoms.

It is important for parents, caregivers, and educators to be aware of the potential impact of depression on children and adolescents and to seek professional help if they suspect a child or adolescent may be experiencing depression. With proper diagnosis and treatment, depression can be effectively managed and treated, and children and adolescents can lead healthy and fulfilling lives.

1. Impact on emotional well-being

Depression can have a profound impact on the emotional well-being of children and adolescents. They may experience persistent feelings of sadness, hopelessness, and worthlessness, which can affect their overall outlook on life. They may have a negative self-image and feel like they are not good enough, leading to a lack of confidence and low self-esteem.

Depression can also lead to a loss of interest or pleasure in activities that the child or adolescent once enjoyed, such as sports, hobbies, or spending time with friends. They may feel isolated and disconnected from others, leading to feelings of loneliness and despair.

In addition to these emotional symptoms, depression can also cause physical symptoms, such as fatigue, changes in appetite and sleep patterns, and physical aches and pains. These symptoms can further impact the emotional well-being of the child or adolescent, as they may feel like they are unable to participate in normal activities or enjoy life.

It is important for parents, caregivers, and educators to be aware of the emotional impact of depression on children and adolescents and to seek professional help if they suspect a child or adolescent may be experiencing depression. With proper diagnosis and treatment, depression can be effectively managed and treated, and children and adolescents can lead healthy and fulfilling lives.

2. Impact on academic performance

Depression can have a significant impact on the academic performance of children and adolescents. Children and adolescents with depression may have difficulty concentrating, remembering things, and completing tasks. They may also have difficulty getting motivated to attend school or complete schoolwork.

Depression can lead to absenteeism from school, tardiness, or a decline in academic performance. They may also have trouble participating in class, engaging in discussions, or collaborating with peers.

Depression can also impact a child or adolescent's ability to think critically and solve problems. They may have negative thoughts about themselves and their abilities, which can impact their self-confidence and their ability to succeed academically.

It is important for parents, caregivers, and educators to be aware of the impact of depression on academic performance and to seek professional help if they suspect a child or adolescent may be experiencing depression. With proper diagnosis and treatment, depression can be effectively managed and treated, and children and adolescents can succeed academically. Additionally, accommodations can be made to support the child or adolescent's academic needs during their recovery period.

3. Impact on social relationships

Depression can have a significant impact on the social relationships of children and adolescents. Children and adolescents with depression may have difficulty making and maintaining friendships, participating in social activities, or engaging with peers. They may feel isolated, disconnected, or lonely, which can lead to further feelings of depression and exacerbate the problem.

Depression can also impact a child or adolescent's family relationships. They may have trouble communicating with their parents or siblings, or they may withdraw from family activities. They may become irritable or easily frustrated, which can lead to conflict within the family.

In addition, depression can impact a child or adolescent's romantic relationships as they get older. They may have trouble forming romantic relationships or maintaining them due to their symptoms of depression.

It is important for parents, caregivers, and educators to be aware of the impact of depression on social relationships and to seek professional help if they suspect a child or adolescent may be experiencing depression. With proper diagnosis and treatment, depression can be effectively managed and treated, and children and adolescents can form healthy social relationships. Additionally, therapy can help children and adolescents develop social skills and cope with any social anxiety or difficulties they may be experiencing.

4. Impact on physical health

Depression can also have a significant impact on the physical health of children and adolescents. Children and adolescents with depression may experience physical symptoms such as headaches, stomachaches, and fatigue. They may also have trouble sleeping or experience changes in appetite, which can impact their overall health and well-being.

Additionally, depression can impact a child or adolescent's overall health behaviors. They may be less likely to engage in physical activity or may have poor eating habits, which can lead to other health problems such as obesity or chronic diseases.

Depression can also impact a child or adolescent's immune system, making them more susceptible to illness or infections. It can also impact their ability to recover from illness or injury, as depression can affect their body's ability to heal and repair itself.

It is important for parents, caregivers, and educators to be aware of the impact of depression on physical health and to seek professional help if they suspect a child or adolescent may be experiencing depression. With proper diagnosis and treatment, depression can be effectively managed and treated, and children and adolescents can improve their overall physical health and well-being. Additionally, therapy can help children and adolescents develop healthy coping mechanisms and self-care habits to support their physical health.

VI. Treatment of Depression in Children and Adolescents

Treatment for depression in children and adolescents typically involves a combination of psychotherapy and medication. The specific treatment plan will depend on the severity of the depression, the age and developmental stage of the child or adolescent, and any underlying medical conditions.

Psychotherapy: Psychotherapy, or talk therapy, is a common and effective treatment for depression in children and adolescents. A trained mental health professional, such as a psychologist or licensed clinical social worker, can work with the child or adolescent to identify and address the underlying causes of their depression. Therapy can help children and adolescents develop coping skills, improve their mood and behavior, and enhance their self-esteem and social skills.

Medication: In some cases, medication may be necessary to treat depression in children and adolescents. Antidepressant medications, such as selective serotonin reuptake inhibitors (SSRIs), can help regulate brain chemicals that are involved in mood regulation. However, these medications should only be used under the close supervision of a healthcare professional, as they can have side effects and may interact with other medications or supplements.

Other therapies: In addition to psychotherapy and medication, there are several other therapies that may be helpful in treating depression in children and adolescents. For example, cognitive-behavioral therapy (CBT) can help children and adolescents identify and challenge negative thought patterns that contribute to their depression. Family therapy can help improve family communication and relationships, which can support the child or adolescent's mental health. Additionally, alternative therapies such as yoga, mindfulness, and art therapy may be helpful in reducing stress and improving mood.

It is important for parents, caregivers, and educators to seek professional help if they suspect a child or adolescent may be experiencing depression. With proper diagnosis and treatment, depression can be effectively managed and treated, and children and adolescents can improve their overall mental health and well-being.

1. Overview of treatment options

The treatment options for depression depend on the severity of the condition and the individual's specific needs. Here is an overview of some of the treatment options available for depression:

1. **Psychotherapy:** Psychotherapy, also known as talk therapy, involves working with a trained mental health professional to identify and address the underlying causes of depression. There are several types of psychotherapy that may be used, such as cognitive-behavioral therapy (CBT), interpersonal therapy, and psychodynamic therapy.

2. **Medication:** Antidepressant medication, such as selective serotonin reuptake inhibitors (SSRIs), can be effective in treating depression by balancing brain chemicals that are involved in mood regulation. However, medication should be used under the close supervision of a healthcare professional, as they can have side effects and may interact with other medications or supplements.

3. **Brain stimulation therapies:** Brain stimulation therapies, such as electroconvulsive therapy (ECT) and transcranial magnetic stimulation (TMS), may be used to treat severe depression when other treatments have not been effective.

4. **Lifestyle changes:** Lifestyle changes can also help manage depression symptoms. For example, regular exercise, healthy eating, and getting enough sleep can improve overall mental health.

5. **Alternative therapies:** Alternative therapies, such as acupuncture, massage, and meditation, may also be used to manage depression symptoms.

It's important to work with a healthcare professional to develop an individualized treatment plan that addresses the specific needs of the individual. Treatment may involve a combination of different therapies to effectively manage depression symptoms.

2. Cognitive-behavioral therapy (CBT)

Cognitive-behavioral therapy (CBT) is a form of psychotherapy that has been shown to be effective in treating depression in children and adolescents. CBT is based on the idea that negative thoughts, feelings, and behaviors can contribute to depression, and that changing these patterns can improve mood and overall well-being.

In CBT, the therapist works with the child or adolescent to identify negative thought patterns and beliefs that may be contributing to their depression. The therapist then helps the individual to challenge and change these negative patterns by providing coping skills and strategies to manage negative thoughts and emotions.

CBT can be delivered in individual or group settings, and typically involves weekly sessions over a period of several months. Homework assignments may also be given to reinforce the skills and strategies learned in therapy.

Research has shown that CBT can be an effective treatment for depression in children and adolescents, and may be used in combination with other treatments, such as medication, for more severe cases. It's important to work with a qualified mental health professional who has experience in treating depression in children and adolescents to ensure the most effective treatment plan.

3. Interpersonal therapy (IPT)

Interpersonal therapy (IPT) is another form of psychotherapy that can be effective in treating depression in children and adolescents. IPT focuses on improving social relationships and addressing interpersonal problems that may be contributing to the child's depression.

In IPT, the therapist works with the child or adolescent to identify specific interpersonal problems that may be contributing to their depression, such as difficulties in communication, conflict with family members or friends, or isolation from social activities. The therapist then helps the child or adolescent to develop skills to improve these relationships and address the underlying issues.

IPT is typically delivered in weekly individual sessions over a period of several months. The therapy is goal-oriented and time-limited, with a focus on addressing the specific interpersonal problems identified by the child or adolescent.

Research has shown that IPT can be an effective treatment for depression in children and adolescents, particularly when combined with other treatments, such as medication or CBT. It's important to work with a qualified mental health professional who has experience in treating depression in children and adolescents to ensure the most effective treatment plan.

4. Medication

Medication can be an effective treatment for depression in children and adolescents, particularly in cases of moderate to severe depression that may not respond to psychotherapy alone. Antidepressant medications work by affecting the levels of certain brain chemicals, such as serotonin and norepinephrine, which are involved in regulating mood.

Selective serotonin reuptake inhibitors (SSRIs) are commonly prescribed antidepressant medications for children and adolescents, as they have been shown to be effective and generally well-tolerated. However, it's important to note that antidepressant medications can have side effects, and there is a potential risk of increased suicidal thoughts or behavior, particularly in younger individuals.

It's important for children and adolescents to be closely monitored by a qualified mental health professional when taking antidepressant medications, and any potential side effects or changes in mood or behavior should be reported immediately.

Medication should be used in combination with psychotherapy, such as CBT or IPT, for the most effective treatment of depression in children and adolescents. It's important to work with a qualified mental health professional who has experience in treating depression in children and adolescents to ensure the most effective treatment plan.

5. Family therapy

Family therapy is another treatment option for depression in children and adolescents. Family therapy involves working with the entire family to address the child's depression and any other family-related issues that may be contributing to the child's symptoms.

In family therapy, the therapist works with the family to identify and address specific issues that may be contributing to the child's depression, such as communication difficulties, conflict, or stress within the family system. The therapist may also work with the family to improve parenting skills or to develop more effective coping strategies.

Family therapy can be particularly effective for younger children, as it allows the child to remain in their familiar environment while working on improving their mental health. It can also be beneficial for adolescents, as it allows for the involvement of the family in the treatment process, which can improve treatment adherence and outcomes.

Research has shown that family therapy can be an effective treatment for depression in children and adolescents, particularly when combined with other treatments, such as medication or individual therapy. It's important to work with a qualified mental health professional who has experience in treating depression in children and adolescents to ensure the most effective treatment plan.

V. Prevention of Depression in Children and Adolescents

Prevention of depression in children and adolescents is an important aspect of mental health care. It involves identifying and addressing risk factors before the onset of depression, as well as promoting protective factors that can help prevent the development of depression.

Here are some strategies for preventing depression in children and adolescents:

1. Building resilience: Encourage children to develop positive coping skills, such as problem-solving and emotion regulation, which can help them better navigate difficult situations.
2. Encouraging physical activity: Regular physical activity has been shown to have a positive effect on mood and can help prevent the development of depression.
3. Teaching social skills: Social support is important for mental health, so teaching children social skills can help them build positive relationships and feel supported.
4. Promoting healthy sleep habits: Adequate sleep is important for mental health, so promoting healthy sleep habits can help prevent the development of depression.
5. Addressing family conflict: Addressing any family-related issues, such as conflict or stress, can help prevent depression in children and adolescents.
6. Reducing stress: Encourage children to engage in stress-reducing activities, such as mindfulness or relaxation exercises.
7. Monitoring for signs of depression: Parents, caregivers, and teachers should be aware of the signs of depression and seek help if they suspect a child is struggling with depression.

By addressing risk factors and promoting protective factors, it is possible to prevent depression in children and adolescents. It is important to seek the help of a mental health professional if a child is showing signs of depression, as early intervention can lead to better outcomes.

1. Early intervention strategies

Early intervention strategies for depression in children and adolescents are important for preventing the onset of more severe symptoms and improving outcomes. Here are some strategies for early intervention:

1. Screening: Regular screening for depression can help identify symptoms early on and provide opportunities for intervention. This can be done in a variety of settings, such as primary care or schools.
2. Psychoeducation: Providing information about depression and its symptoms can help individuals identify and understand their own experiences. This can also help reduce stigma and increase help-seeking behaviors.
3. Cognitive-behavioral therapy (CBT): CBT is an evidence-based treatment that has been shown to be effective in treating depression in children and adolescents. Early intervention with CBT can prevent symptoms from worsening and reduce the risk of long-term problems.
4. Family therapy: Family therapy can help address family-related issues that may contribute to depression in children and adolescents. Early intervention with family therapy can improve family functioning and prevent symptoms from worsening.
5. Medication: In some cases, medication may be necessary to treat depression in children and adolescents. Early intervention with medication can prevent symptoms from worsening and improve outcomes.
6. Supportive interventions: Providing support and encouragement to children and adolescents can help prevent symptoms from worsening and promote recovery. This can include providing emotional support, helping with problem-solving, and encouraging positive coping strategies.

Early intervention is crucial for preventing depression in children and adolescents from developing into more severe mental health problems. By addressing symptoms early on, individuals can receive the support and treatment they need to improve their mental health and well-being.

2. Promoting resilience and coping skills

Promoting resilience and coping skills is an important aspect of preventing depression in children and adolescents. Here are some strategies for promoting resilience and coping skills:

1. Building strong relationships: Having supportive relationships with family, friends, and peers can provide a sense of belonging and support during difficult times.
2. Developing problem-solving skills: Encouraging children and adolescents to identify and solve problems can help them feel more confident in their ability to handle challenges.
3. Encouraging positive self-talk: Helping children and adolescents identify and challenge negative thoughts and replace them with positive self-talk can improve their self-esteem and confidence.
4. Promoting healthy lifestyle habits: Encouraging healthy habits such as regular exercise, good nutrition, and adequate sleep can improve mental health and well-being.
5. Teaching stress management skills: Helping children and adolescents develop skills to manage stress, such as relaxation techniques, mindfulness, or breathing exercises, can improve their ability to cope with challenging situations.
6. Building a sense of purpose: Encouraging children and adolescents to pursue activities and hobbies that provide a sense of purpose and meaning can improve their overall sense of well-being.

By promoting resilience and coping skills, children and adolescents can develop the tools they need to handle life's challenges and prevent depression from taking hold. Encouraging healthy habits, building strong relationships, and teaching stress management skills are all key components of promoting resilience and well-being.

• • • •

3. REDUCING RISK FACTORS

Reducing risk factors can also help prevent depression in children and adolescents. Here are some strategies for reducing risk factors:

1. Addressing family dysfunction: Family dysfunction, such as conflict or abuse, can increase the risk of depression in children and adolescents. Addressing and resolving family issues can reduce this risk.
2. Providing a safe and supportive environment: A safe and supportive environment can help children and adolescents feel secure and reduce the risk of depression. This can include providing a stable home environment, having clear and consistent rules and boundaries, and providing emotional support.
3. Addressing trauma: Exposure to trauma, such as abuse, neglect, or violence, can increase the risk of depression. Addressing and treating trauma can reduce this risk.
4. Addressing academic stress: Academic stress can increase the risk of depression in children and adolescents. Providing academic support and resources, such as tutoring or counseling, can help reduce this stress.
5. Reducing exposure to media: Exposure to violent or negative media can increase the risk of depression. Limiting exposure to negative media and promoting positive media can reduce this risk.

By addressing risk factors, children and adolescents can have a lower risk of developing depression. Providing a safe and supportive environment, addressing family dysfunction, and reducing exposure to media are all key strategies for reducing risk factors.

<u>4. Encouraging healthy lifestyles</u>

Encouraging healthy lifestyles can also play an important role in preventing depression in children and adolescents. Here are some ways to promote healthy lifestyles:

1. Encouraging physical activity: Regular physical activity has been shown to improve mood and reduce the risk of depression. Encourage children and adolescents to participate in physical activities they enjoy, such as sports or dance.
2. Promoting healthy eating habits: A healthy diet can also help reduce the risk of depression. Encourage children and adolescents to eat a balanced diet with plenty of fruits, vegetables, whole grains, and lean

protein.

3. Getting enough sleep: Adequate sleep is important for both physical and emotional health. Encourage children and adolescents to get enough sleep each night by establishing a regular sleep routine and minimizing screen time before bed.
4. Limiting screen time: Excessive screen time has been linked to depression in children and adolescents. Encourage children and adolescents to limit their screen time and engage in other activities, such as reading or playing outside.
5. Building social connections: Social support is important for emotional well-being. Encourage children and adolescents to build and maintain social connections with friends and family members.

By promoting healthy lifestyles, children and adolescents can have a lower risk of depression. Encouraging physical activity, healthy eating habits, adequate sleep, and social connections can all help reduce the risk of depression.

VI. Supporting a Child or Adolescent with Depression

Supporting a child or adolescent with depression can be challenging, but it is important to provide them with love, understanding, and guidance. Here are some ways to support a child or adolescent with depression:

1. Educate yourself: Learn as much as you can about depression in children and adolescents, including its symptoms, causes, and treatments. This will help you better understand what your child or adolescent is going through and how you can help.
2. Communicate openly: Encourage your child or adolescent to talk about their feelings and listen to what they have to say without judgment or criticism. Offer reassurance and support, and let them know that it is okay to ask for help.
3. Provide a stable and supportive environment: Try to create a stable and supportive environment at home by establishing routines, setting clear expectations, and providing opportunities for positive interactions with family and friends.
4. Seek professional help: If your child or adolescent is experiencing severe depression or suicidal thoughts, seek professional help immediately. A mental health professional can provide a proper diagnosis and recommend appropriate treatment.
5. Encourage self-care: Encourage your child or adolescent to engage in self-care activities, such as exercise, relaxation techniques, and hobbies. These activities can help improve their mood and reduce stress.
6. Advocate for them: If your child or adolescent needs additional support at school or in other settings, advocate for their needs and work with teachers and other professionals to ensure they receive the necessary accommodations and support.

Supporting a child or adolescent with depression can be challenging, but with love, understanding, and guidance, you can help them manage their symptoms and improve their emotional well-being.

1. Communicating with children and adolescents about depression

Communicating with children and adolescents about depression is an important aspect of supporting them. Here is an outline of what can be included in a book chapter on this topic:

I. Importance of communication

1. The importance of open communication in supporting a child or adolescent with depression
2. Common misconceptions about discussing mental health with children and adolescents

II. How to talk to children and adolescents about depression

1. Choosing the right time and place to have the conversation
2. Age-appropriate language and concepts to use
3. Encouraging children and adolescents to express themselves and their feelings
4. Active listening and validating their experiences
5. Addressing any concerns or questions they may have

III. What to say and what not to say

1. Words and phrases that can be helpful and supportive
2. Words and phrases that can be harmful or dismissive
3. Strategies for responding to difficult questions or statements

IV. Discussing treatment options

1. Explaining the different types of treatment available
2. Addressing any concerns or fears they may have about treatment
3. Involving them in the decision-making process as appropriate

V. Maintaining ongoing communication

1. The importance of ongoing conversations about mental health
2. Strategies for maintaining open communication over time
3. Signs to look out for that may indicate the need for additional support or intervention

VI. Supporting the child or adolescent's emotional well-being

1. Strategies for promoting emotional well-being, such as self-care, mindfulness, and positive coping strategies
2. Encouraging social support and connecting with others who may be experiencing similar challenges

VII. Seeking additional support as needed

1. The importance of seeking additional support from mental health professionals or other resources when necessary
2. Strategies for identifying when additional support may be needed and where to turn for help.

2.Providing emotional support

Providing Emotional Support for Children and Adolescents with Depression

Depression is a challenging condition that can have a significant impact on children and adolescents. When someone you care about is struggling with depression, it can be difficult to know how to provide the emotional support they need. However, with the right strategies and approach, you can help your loved one manage their depression and improve their emotional well-being.

Section 1: Understanding the Emotional Impact of Depression on Children and Adolescents

1. Depression can have a significant impact on the emotional well-being of children and adolescents. They may experience feelings of sadness, hopelessness, and worthlessness. They may also feel anxious, irritable, and have difficulty concentrating.
2. It is important to understand that depression is an illness and not a personal weakness or character flaw. Children and adolescents may need support and reassurance to overcome any feelings of shame or stigma they may have associated with their depression.

Section 2: Building a Supportive Relationship

1. Building a supportive relationship with a child or adolescent with depression is essential for providing emotional support. Listen actively and show empathy for their experience, and try to understand what they are going through.

2. Encourage them to express their feelings and provide a safe space for them to do so. Acknowledge their emotions and validate their experiences, even if you cannot fully understand them.

Section 3: Offering Practical Support

1. Depression can make everyday tasks feel overwhelming. Offering practical support can help a child or adolescent with depression manage their daily responsibilities and feel more in control of their life. This can include helping with homework, cooking a meal, or running errands.
2. Encourage them to engage in activities they enjoy, and offer to participate in these activities with them. This can help them feel more connected and supported.

Section 4: Promoting Self-Care

1. Self-care is an essential part of managing depression. Encourage a child or adolescent with depression to take care of themselves physically and mentally. This can include getting enough sleep, eating healthy foods, and engaging in physical activity.
2. Encourage them to engage in activities that promote relaxation and stress relief, such as mindfulness exercises, deep breathing, or yoga.

Section 5: Seeking Professional Help

1. It is important to seek professional help for a child or adolescent with depression. A mental health professional can provide additional support and guidance, and may recommend therapy or medication to manage their symptoms.
2. Help them schedule appointments and offer to accompany them to their appointments if they would like support.

Providing emotional support for a child or adolescent with depression can be challenging, but it is essential for their emotional well-being. By building a supportive relationship, offering practical support, promoting self-care, and seeking professional help, you can help them manage their depression and improve their quality of life.

3. Supporting treatment plans

Supporting treatment plans for children and adolescents with depression involves a number of strategies, such as:

1. Encouraging treatment compliance: It is important to encourage the child or adolescent to adhere to their treatment plan, which may include medication, therapy, or a combination of both.
2. Providing transportation: It can be helpful to provide transportation to appointments and ensure that the child or adolescent has the necessary resources to attend therapy sessions and take medication as prescribed.
3. Creating a supportive environment: Creating a supportive and understanding environment at home and school can help the child or adolescent feel more comfortable discussing their struggles and progress with depression.
4. Educating oneself: Educating oneself on depression and its treatment can help parents or caregivers better understand the child or adolescent's experiences and provide more effective support.
5. Seeking support for oneself: Caring for a child or adolescent with depression can be emotionally taxing, and seeking support for oneself can help prevent caregiver burnout.

6. Encouraging healthy habits: Encouraging healthy habits such as regular exercise, healthy eating, and adequate sleep can help improve overall well-being and may also have a positive impact on depression symptoms.

7. Promoting social connections: Encouraging the child or adolescent to participate in social activities and hobbies can promote positive social connections and help counteract feelings of isolation that may be associated with depression.

<u>4. Advocating for the child or adolescent</u>

Parents or caregivers can play a critical role in advocating for their child or adolescent with depression. The following are some strategies that may be helpful:

1. Educate yourself: Learn about depression and the available treatment options. Understand the rights of your child in the educational system and how to navigate the mental health system.

2. Build a support network: Seek out support from other parents or caregivers who have dealt with similar challenges. Joining a support group or seeking out therapy for yourself can also be helpful.

3. Communicate with the school: Talk to your child's teachers and school counselor about your child's depression and how it may be affecting their academic performance. Work with the school to develop a plan for accommodations or modifications, such as extra time on assignments or a reduced workload.

4. Advocate for mental health services: If your child needs mental health services, work with your insurance company or healthcare provider to access the necessary care. If you encounter barriers, consider reaching out to a mental health advocacy organization for assistance.

5. Stay informed and involved: Stay up-to-date on your child's treatment plan and attend appointments with them. Be an active participant in their care and advocate for their needs.

6. Address stigma: Educate others about depression and work to reduce stigma. Encourage your child to talk openly about their experiences and advocate for themselves.

By advocating for your child or adolescent with depression, you can help ensure that they receive the care and support they need to thrive.

VII. Challenges and Controversies in Treating Depression in Children and Adolescents

Treating depression in children and adolescents can present unique challenges and controversies. One challenge is accurately diagnosing depression in this population, as symptoms may be different from those seen in adults and can often be mistaken for typical teenage behavior. Additionally, children and adolescents may not have the ability to articulate their emotions or may not want to express them, making diagnosis and treatment difficult.

Another challenge is determining the most effective treatment approach for this population. While medication and therapy are commonly used treatments, there is controversy surrounding the use of antidepressants in children and adolescents due to potential side effects and concerns about long-term effects on brain development. There is also debate about the most effective type of therapy, as different approaches may be more or less effective depending on the individual.

Another controversial topic is the role of parents and caregivers in the treatment process. While involving parents in treatment can be beneficial, some argue that over-involvement can lead to negative outcomes and hinder the adolescent's independence and development. Additionally, there may be cultural differences in beliefs about mental health and treatment that can affect the approach to treating depression in children and adolescents.

Overall, addressing these challenges and controversies requires ongoing research and collaboration between mental health professionals, patients, and families. By continuing to explore new treatment options and addressing concerns around current approaches, we can work towards better outcomes for children and adolescents living with depression.

1. Controversies surrounding medication use in children and adolescents

The use of medication in the treatment of depression in children and adolescents is a controversial issue. Some of the controversies surrounding medication use include:

1. **Safety concerns:** Antidepressant medications have been linked to an increased risk of suicidal ideation and behavior in children and adolescents. This has led to warnings from regulatory agencies and cautious prescribing practices by healthcare providers.

2. **Efficacy concerns:** Studies have shown that antidepressant medications may not be as effective in treating depression in children and adolescents as they are in adults. Additionally, there is concern that the benefits of medication may be outweighed by the potential risks.

3. **Side effects:** Antidepressant medications can cause a range of side effects, including nausea, dizziness, weight gain, and sexual dysfunction. Children and adolescents may be particularly vulnerable to these side effects.

4. **Stigma:** There is still a significant amount of stigma associated with mental health disorders and their treatment. Some parents may be hesitant to have their child take medication for fear of being seen as a "bad parent" or because of concerns about the stigma associated with mental health treatment.

5. **Long-term effects:** There is limited research on the long-term effects of antidepressant medication use in children and adolescents. Some experts are concerned that the use of medication may interfere with normal brain development or have other long-term effects on physical and mental health.

It is important for healthcare providers and families to carefully consider the potential benefits and risks of medication use in the treatment of depression in children and adolescents, and to make treatment decisions based on the individual needs of the child or adolescent.

<u>2. Challenges in identifying and treating depression in children and adolescents</u>

Identifying and treating depression in children and adolescents can present several challenges. Some of these challenges include:

1. **Difficulty in recognizing symptoms:** Children and adolescents may not have the vocabulary to express how they are feeling or may not understand their emotions. This can make it challenging for parents and healthcare providers to identify symptoms of depression.
2. **Stigma and shame:** Children and adolescents may feel ashamed or embarrassed about their feelings and may not seek help or disclose their symptoms.
3. **Co-occurring conditions:** Children and adolescents with depression often have co-occurring conditions, such as anxiety or ADHD, which can complicate treatment.
4. **Limited treatment options:** There are fewer treatment options for children and adolescents with depression compared to adults. Some medications and therapies may not be suitable or approved for use in children and adolescents.
5. **Parental involvement:** Treatment often requires parental involvement, which can be challenging if the parent is also struggling with mental health issues or if the parent is resistant to seeking help.
6. **<u>Compliance with treatment:</u>** Children and adolescents may have difficulty adhering to treatment plans due to lack of motivation, forgetfulness, or other factors.

Addressing these challenges requires a comprehensive approach that involves the child or adolescent, their family, healthcare providers, and the community. It is important to create a supportive environment that promotes mental health and encourages open communication about mental health issues.

<u>VIII. Understanding Depression and Anxiety</u>

Depression and anxiety are two mental health disorders that can have a significant impact on an individual's emotional, cognitive, and physical functioning. While they are distinct conditions, they often coexist and can have similar symptoms. Understanding the characteristics of depression and anxiety is essential in recognizing the need for treatment and developing effective strategies for managing these conditions.

Depression is a mood disorder characterized by persistent feelings of sadness, hopelessness, and loss of interest in activities that were once pleasurable. Other common symptoms of depression may include:

1. Changes in appetite and weight
2. Difficulty sleeping or oversleeping
3. Fatigue or loss of energy
4. Difficulty concentrating or making decisions
5. Thoughts of death or suicide

Anxiety, on the other hand, involves excessive worry and fear about everyday situations or events, and can lead to physical symptoms such as sweating, rapid heartbeat, and difficulty breathing. Some common symptoms of anxiety include:

1. Restlessness or feeling on edge
2. Irritability
3. Difficulty concentrating
4. Muscle tension
5. Avoidance of certain situations or activities

While depression and anxiety are separate disorders, they can coexist and even reinforce each other. For example, someone with depression may also experience anxiety as a symptom of their depression, while someone with anxiety may develop depression as a result of their constant worrying and fear.

It is important to note that depression and anxiety are treatable conditions, and a mental health professional can help develop a personalized treatment plan that addresses both conditions if they coexist. With proper treatment and support, it is possible to manage depression and anxiety and improve overall well-being.

1. Definition and explanation of depression and anxiety

Depression and anxiety are two common mental health conditions that can affect an individual's thoughts, emotions, and behaviors. Although they share some similarities, they are distinct conditions with different symptoms and causes.

Depression is a mood disorder characterized by persistent feelings of sadness, hopelessness, and loss of interest or pleasure in activities that were once enjoyable. Other symptoms of depression may include changes in appetite or weight, difficulty sleeping or oversleeping, fatigue, difficulty concentrating, and thoughts of death or suicide. Depression can range in severity from mild to severe and can significantly impact an individual's daily functioning.

Anxiety, on the other hand, is a mental health condition characterized by excessive worry or fear about everyday situations or events. Anxiety can manifest in physical symptoms such as sweating, rapid heartbeat, and difficulty breathing, and can interfere with an individual's ability to carry out daily activities. Common types of anxiety disorders include generalized anxiety disorder, panic disorder, social anxiety disorder, and specific phobias.

The causes of depression and anxiety can vary, but they often involve a combination of genetic, environmental, and psychological factors. For example, a family history of depression or anxiety may increase an individual's risk for developing these conditions, as can experiencing traumatic or stressful life events. Certain medical conditions, such as thyroid disorders, can also contribute to the development of depression and anxiety.

While depression and anxiety can be challenging conditions to live with, they are treatable with the help of mental health professionals. Treatment options may include therapy, medication, lifestyle changes, and self-care strategies such as exercise and mindfulness practices. Early intervention and ongoing support can help individuals manage their symptoms and improve their overall quality of life.

2. Symptoms and diagnosis criteria

The symptoms of depression and anxiety can vary from person to person, but there are specific diagnostic criteria that mental health professionals use to identify these conditions.

Symptoms of Depression:

To meet the criteria for a diagnosis of depression, an individual must have experienced at least five of the following symptoms for a period of at least two weeks, and they must represent a change from their previous functioning. One of the symptoms must be either persistent feelings of sadness or loss of interest in previously enjoyed activities.

The symptoms include:

1. Persistent feelings of sadness, hopelessness, or emptiness
2. Loss of interest or pleasure in activities that were once enjoyable
3. Changes in appetite and weight
4. Difficulty sleeping or oversleeping
5. Fatigue or loss of energy
6. Feelings of worthlessness or excessive guilt
7. Difficulty concentrating or making decisions
8. Thoughts of death or suicide

Symptoms of Anxiety:

To meet the criteria for a diagnosis of an anxiety disorder, an individual must experience excessive worry or fear about everyday situations or events, along with physical symptoms such as sweating, rapid heartbeat, and difficulty breathing. The specific symptoms depend on the type of anxiety disorder, but **common symptoms include:**

1. Restlessness or feeling on edge
2. Irritability
3. Difficulty concentrating
4. Muscle tension
5. Avoidance of certain situations or activities

Diagnosis:

A diagnosis of depression or anxiety is typically made by a mental health professional, such as a psychiatrist or psychologist. To diagnose depression or anxiety, the professional will typically conduct a clinical interview and may use standardized assessments to evaluate the severity and duration of symptoms.

It is important to note that a diagnosis of depression or anxiety requires careful consideration of an individual's symptoms and overall functioning, and it should only be made by a trained mental health professional. If you or someone you know is experiencing symptoms of depression or anxiety, seeking professional help is important to receive proper diagnosis and treatment.

3. Prevalence of the conditions

Depression and anxiety are two of the most common mental health conditions in the world, affecting millions of people of all ages, genders, and cultural backgrounds.

Prevalence of Depression:

According to the World Health Organization (WHO), depression is the leading cause of disability worldwide, affecting over 264 million people globally. In the United States alone, approximately 7% of adults experience at least one major depressive episode in a given year, with women being more likely to be affected than men. Depression can occur at any age, but it often first presents in young adulthood.

Prevalence of Anxiety:

Anxiety disorders are also highly prevalent, affecting an estimated 284 million people worldwide, according to the WHO. In the United States, anxiety disorders are the most common mental health condition, with approximately 31% of adults experiencing an anxiety disorder at some point in their lives. Women are also more likely to be affected by anxiety disorders than men.

Comorbidity:

It is important to note that depression and anxiety often co-occur, with research suggesting that up to 60% of individuals with depression also have symptoms of anxiety, and vice versa. This comorbidity can complicate diagnosis and treatment, and it highlights the importance of a comprehensive assessment by a mental health professional.

It is important to remember that depression and anxiety are treatable conditions, and seeking professional help can be the first step towards managing symptoms and improving overall quality of life.

IX. Supporting a Loved One with Depression and Anxiety

Supporting a loved one with depression and anxiety can be challenging, but it is essential to help them navigate their symptoms and seek appropriate treatment. Here are some tips for supporting a loved one with depression and anxiety:

1. Educate yourself about depression and anxiety: Learn as much as you can about these conditions, including their symptoms, causes, and treatment options. This will help you understand what your loved one is going through and how you can support them.

2. Encourage your loved one to seek professional help: Mental health professionals can provide a range of treatments for depression and anxiety, including medication, therapy, and other supportive interventions. Encourage your loved one to seek help from a qualified mental health professional, and offer to help them find a provider if needed.

3. Listen without judgment: When your loved one wants to talk about their feelings and experiences, listen attentively and without judgment. Avoid offering unsolicited advice or minimizing their feelings, and let them know that you are there to support them.

4. Be patient: Recovery from depression and anxiety can be a slow and difficult process, and there may be setbacks along the way. Be patient with your loved one and offer ongoing support and encouragement.

5. Help your loved one practice self-care: Encourage your loved one to prioritize self-care activities, such as exercise, healthy eating, and stress management techniques. Offer to participate in these activities with them and provide practical support, such as helping them prepare healthy meals or going for a walk together.

6. Take care of yourself: Supporting a loved one with depression and anxiety can be emotionally taxing, so it is essential to prioritize your own self-care. Make sure you are taking care of your own physical and emotional needs, and seek support from friends, family, or a mental health professional if needed.

Supporting a loved one with depression and anxiety can be challenging, but with patience, understanding, and appropriate support, you can help them navigate their symptoms and work towards recovery.

1. Strategies for supporting a loved one with depression and anxiety

Here are some strategies that can help you support a loved one with depression and anxiety:

1. Offer emotional support: One of the most important things you can do for your loved one is to offer emotional support. This includes listening without judgment, expressing empathy, and offering words of encouragement.
2. Encourage them to seek professional help: It is important for your loved one to seek professional help from a mental health professional, such as a therapist or psychiatrist. Encourage them to make an appointment and offer to help them find a provider if needed.
3. Help them stick to their treatment plan: If your loved one is receiving treatment for depression or anxiety, help them stick to their treatment plan. This may include reminding them to take their medication, attending therapy sessions with them, or helping them practice self-care.
4. Learn about their condition: Educate yourself about your loved one's condition and its symptoms. This will help you understand what they are going through and how you can best support them.
5. Help them practice self-care: Encourage your loved one to practice self-care activities, such as exercise, healthy eating, and stress management techniques. Offer to participate in these activities with them and provide practical support, such as helping them prepare healthy meals or going for a walk together.
6. Be patient and understanding: Recovery from depression and anxiety can be a slow process, and there may be setbacks along the way. Be patient and understanding, and offer ongoing support and encouragement.
7. Take care of yourself: Supporting a loved one with depression and

anxiety can be emotionally taxing. It is important to take care of yourself and seek support from friends, family, or a mental health professional if needed.

Remember that everyone's experience with depression and anxiety is unique, and what works for one person may not work for another. Be flexible and willing to try different strategies to support your loved one on their journey to recovery.

2. Understanding their experiences and needs

Understanding your loved one's experiences and needs is crucial to supporting them effectively. Here are some tips to help you better understand your loved one:

1. Listen attentively: When your loved one wants to talk about their experiences with depression and anxiety, listen attentively and without judgment. Allow them to express their feelings and experiences in their own words.

2. Ask questions: If you are unsure about something, ask your loved one questions to clarify. This will help you better understand their experiences and needs.

3. Learn about their condition: Educate yourself about your loved one's condition and its symptoms. This will help you understand what they are going through and how you can best support them.

4. Respect their boundaries: Your loved one may not want to talk about their experiences with depression and anxiety all the time. Respect their boundaries and let them know that you are there for them when they are ready to talk.

5. Be compassionate: Show your loved one compassion and empathy. Let them know that you care about them and are there to support them.

6. Support their treatment plan: Encourage your loved one to seek professional help and support them in sticking to their treatment plan. This may include attending therapy sessions with them or helping them practice self-care.

7. Take care of yourself: Supporting a loved one with depression and anxiety can be emotionally taxing. Make sure you take care of yourself and seek support from friends, family, or a mental health professional if

needed.

Remember that everyone's experience with depression and anxiety is unique. By listening, learning, and being compassionate, you can better understand your loved one's experiences and needs, and provide effective support.

3. Coping with caregiver burnout

Caring for a loved one with depression and anxiety can be emotionally taxing and can lead to caregiver burnout. Here are some tips to help cope with caregiver burnout:

1. Take breaks: It is important to take regular breaks from caregiving to prevent burnout. Schedule time for yourself, such as going for a walk or practicing a hobby.
2. Seek support: Seek support from friends, family, or a mental health professional. Talking to someone about your experiences can help you manage stress and prevent burnout.
3. Practice self-care: Practice self-care activities such as exercise, healthy eating, and relaxation techniques. Taking care of yourself can help you manage stress and prevent burnout.
4. Set boundaries: Set boundaries around caregiving, such as limiting the amount of time you spend caregiving each day. This can help prevent burnout and allow you to take care of your own needs.
5. Learn about caregiver resources: There are many resources available to help caregivers, such as support groups and respite care. Learn about these resources and consider utilizing them to help prevent burnout.
6. Take care of your physical health: Taking care of your physical health, such as getting enough sleep and eating a healthy diet, can help you manage stress and prevent burnout.
7. Practice mindfulness: Mindfulness techniques, such as meditation or yoga, can help you manage stress and prevent burnout.

Remember, taking care of yourself is just as important as taking care of your loved one. By practicing self-care, seeking support, and setting boundaries, you can prevent caregiver burnout and provide effective support to your loved one with depression and anxiety.

X. Symptoms of Depression

Depression can present with a range of symptoms, both emotional and physical. The severity and duration of symptoms can vary from person to person. Some common symptoms of depression include:

1. **Emotional symptoms:**

- Persistent feelings of sadness, hopelessness, or emptiness
- Loss of interest or pleasure in activities that were once enjoyable
- Feelings of guilt, worthlessness, or helplessness
- Anxiety, irritability, or restlessness
- Difficulty concentrating, making decisions, or remembering things
- Suicidal thoughts or behaviors

1. **Physical symptoms:**

- Changes in appetite, weight loss or gain
- Insomnia or oversleeping
- Fatigue or loss of energy
- Chronic pain, headaches, or digestive issues

1. **Behavioral symptoms:**

- Avoiding social activities or withdrawing from friends and family
- Decreased productivity or difficulty functioning at work or school
- Substance abuse or engaging in risky behaviors
- Self-harm or suicidal behavior

It is important to note that not all individuals with depression will experience all of these symptoms, and the symptoms may vary in severity and duration. If you or someone you know is experiencing these symptoms, it is important to seek help from a mental health professional.

1. Emotional symptoms

Emotional symptoms are a key feature of depression, and they can have a significant impact on a person's mental and emotional well-being. Some of the emotional symptoms of depression include:

1. Persistent feelings of sadness, hopelessness, or emptiness: Individuals with depression often feel sad or empty for extended periods, even when there is no apparent reason for their mood. These feelings can be intense and overwhelming, leading to a loss of interest in life and difficulty enjoying daily activities.
2. Loss of interest or pleasure in activities that were once enjoyable: Individuals with depression often lose interest in hobbies or activities they once enjoyed, which can further contribute to feelings of sadness and isolation.
3. Feelings of guilt, worthlessness, or helplessness: Depression can lead individuals to feel guilty, worthless, or helpless, even when they have done nothing wrong. These feelings can be pervasive and can lead to low self-esteem and a sense of hopelessness.
4. Anxiety, irritability, or restlessness: Individuals with depression may experience anxiety, irritability, or restlessness. These emotions can be intense and make it difficult to relax or concentrate.
5. Difficulty concentrating, making decisions, or remembering things: Depression can make it challenging for individuals to concentrate, make decisions, or remember important details. This can impact their ability to function at work or school and can further contribute to feelings of frustration and low self-esteem.
6. Suicidal thoughts or behaviors: Individuals with severe depression may experience suicidal thoughts or behaviors. It is essential to seek immediate help if you or someone you know is experiencing suicidal thoughts or engaging in self-harm.

2. Physical symptoms

Depression can also present with a variety of physical symptoms, which can often be challenging to distinguish from other medical conditions. Some common physical symptoms of depression include:

1. Changes in appetite, weight loss or gain: Depression can cause changes in appetite, leading to significant weight loss or gain. Individuals with depression may experience a loss of appetite or find themselves overeating as a way to cope with their emotions.
2. Insomnia or oversleeping: Individuals with depression may experience changes in their sleep patterns, such as insomnia or oversleeping. This can make it difficult to get restful sleep and can impact their energy levels and ability to function during the day.
3. Fatigue or loss of energy: Depression can cause fatigue and a lack of energy, making it challenging to complete daily activities or concentrate.
4. Chronic pain, headaches, or digestive issues: Individuals with depression may experience chronic pain, such as headaches, back pain, or digestive issues. These symptoms can be caused by the physical tension and stress that depression places on the body.

It is important to note that physical symptoms alone are not enough to diagnose depression. However, if these symptoms persist for an extended period and are accompanied by emotional symptoms, it may be a sign of depression. Seeking help from a mental health professional is essential to receive an accurate diagnosis and effective treatment.

3. Behavioral symptoms

Depression can also impact an individual's behavior and the way they interact with others. Some common behavioral symptoms of depression include:

1. Avoiding social activities or withdrawing from friends and family: Depression can cause individuals to feel socially isolated and withdrawn. They may avoid social activities or spend more time alone, which can exacerbate their feelings of loneliness and sadness.
2. Decreased productivity or difficulty functioning at work or school: Individuals with depression may find it challenging to focus or concentrate, impacting their productivity at work or school. They may also struggle to meet deadlines or complete tasks.
3. Substance abuse or engaging in risky behaviors: Depression can lead to substance abuse or engaging in risky behaviors, such as gambling or

unsafe sex. These behaviors may be used as a way to cope with the emotional pain of depression.

4. Self-harm or suicidal behavior: Individuals with severe depression may engage in self-harm or suicidal behavior as a way to cope with their emotions. It is essential to seek immediate help if you or someone you know is experiencing suicidal thoughts or engaging in self-harm.

It is important to note that these behavioral symptoms can have a significant impact on an individual's life and relationships. Seeking help from a mental health professional can provide effective treatment and support to manage these symptoms and improve overall well-being.

XI. Causes of Depression

Depression is a complex mental health condition that can be caused by a combination of biological, environmental, and psychological factors. Here are some common causes of depression:

1. Genetics: Depression can run in families, indicating that there may be a genetic component to the condition.
2. Brain chemistry: Imbalances in neurotransmitters, which are chemicals in the brain that regulate mood, can lead to depression.
3. Environmental factors: Traumatic events, such as abuse, neglect, or the death of a loved one, can trigger depression. Chronic stress, financial problems, or a lack of social support can also contribute to the development of depression.
4. Medical conditions: Certain medical conditions, such as chronic pain, thyroid disorders, or neurological conditions, can increase the risk of depression.
5. Substance abuse: Substance abuse, particularly with drugs that impact mood, can increase the risk of depression.
6. Hormonal changes: Hormonal changes, such as those that occur during pregnancy, menopause, or after giving birth, can lead to depression.

It's important to remember that depression is a complex condition and can be caused by a combination of factors. Seeking help from a mental health professional is essential to receive an accurate diagnosis and effective treatment.

1. Biological factors

Biological factors can contribute to the development of depression, including:

1. Neurotransmitter imbalances: Neurotransmitters are chemicals in the brain that regulate mood, and imbalances in these chemicals can lead to depression. For example, a deficiency in serotonin, a neurotransmitter that regulates mood, has been linked to depression.
2. Genetics: There is evidence that depression can run in families, indicating that there may be a genetic component to the condition.

However, the exact genes that contribute to depression are not yet fully understood.

3. Brain structure and function: Studies have shown that individuals with depression may have differences in the structure and function of certain areas of the brain, particularly those involved in emotional regulation.

4. Hormonal imbalances: Hormonal imbalances, such as those that occur during pregnancy, menopause, or after giving birth, can increase the risk of depression. In addition, thyroid disorders, which can affect hormone levels, have also been linked to depression.

5. Chronic stress: Chronic stress can impact the function of the hypothalamic-pituitary-adrenal (HPA) axis, which regulates the stress response in the body. Changes in the HPA axis can lead to imbalances in neurotransmitters and increase the risk of depression.

It is important to note that biological factors alone are not enough to cause depression, and a combination of genetic, environmental, and psychological factors can contribute to its development. Seeking help from a mental health professional can provide effective treatment and support to manage biological factors that contribute to depression.

2. Psychological factors

Psychological factors can also contribute to the development of depression, including:

1. Negative thought patterns: Negative thought patterns, such as self-criticism or negative self-talk, can contribute to the development of depression. Individuals who have a negative outlook on themselves or their situation may be more prone to depression.

2. Personality traits: Certain personality traits, such as low self-esteem or perfectionism, can increase the risk of depression. Individuals who struggle with these traits may be more likely to experience negative emotions and develop depression.

3. Trauma and stress: Traumatic events, such as abuse or neglect, can increase the risk of depression. Chronic stress, such as financial or relationship problems, can also contribute to the development of

depression.

4. Learned helplessness: Individuals who have experienced repeated failures or negative experiences may develop a sense of learned helplessness, leading to feelings of hopelessness and depression.

5. Interpersonal issues: Relationship problems, such as conflicts with family or friends, can increase the risk of depression. In addition, a lack of social support or feeling isolated can also contribute to the development of depression.

It is important to note that psychological factors are not the sole cause of depression, and a combination of biological, environmental, and psychological factors can contribute to its development. Seeking help from a mental health professional can provide effective treatment and support to manage psychological factors that contribute to depression.

3. Environmental factors

Environmental factors can also contribute to the development of depression, including:

1. **Life events:** Traumatic events, such as the death of a loved one, a serious illness, or a relationship breakup, can trigger depression. In addition, ongoing stressors such as work-related stress, financial difficulties, or relationship problems can also contribute to the development of depression.

2. **Social factors:** A lack of social support or feeling isolated can increase the risk of depression. Individuals who feel disconnected from their family, friends, or community may be more likely to develop depression.

3. **Substance abuse:** Substance abuse, particularly with drugs that impact mood, can increase the risk of depression. Individuals who use substances to cope with stress or difficult emotions may be more prone to depression.

4. **Living environment:** Living in an unsafe or unstable environment can contribute to the development of depression. Individuals who live in poverty, have limited access to resources, or live in unsafe neighborhoods may be at increased risk of depression.

5. **Cultural factors:** Cultural factors, such as discrimination or stigma, can contribute to the development of depression. Individuals who face discrimination or marginalization may be more prone to depression.

It is important to note that environmental factors are not the sole cause of depression, and a combination of biological, environmental, and psychological factors can contribute to its development. Seeking help from a mental health professional can provide effective treatment and support to manage environmental factors that contribute to depression.

XII. <u>Types of Depression</u>

There are several different types of depression, including:

1. Major depression: This is the most common type of depression and is characterized by a persistent feeling of sadness, hopelessness, and a lack of interest or pleasure in activities that were once enjoyable. It can interfere with daily activities and may require treatment.
2. Persistent depressive disorder: This type of depression is characterized by a chronic feeling of sadness and a lack of interest or pleasure in activities for at least two years.
3. Bipolar disorder: This type of depression is characterized by episodes of depression alternating with episodes of mania or hypomania, which are periods of elevated mood, energy, and activity levels.
4. Seasonal affective disorder (SAD): This type of depression is related to changes in the season, typically occurring in the fall or winter months when there is less daylight. It is characterized by symptoms of depression, such as sadness, fatigue, and difficulty concentrating.
5. Psychotic depression: This type of depression is characterized by symptoms of major depression along with psychotic symptoms, such as hallucinations or delusions.
6. Postpartum depression: This type of depression occurs after giving birth and is characterized by feelings of sadness, anxiety, and exhaustion that can interfere with daily activities and caring for the baby.

It is important to note that depression can vary in severity and duration and may require different treatments depending on the type and individual symptoms. Seeking help from a mental health professional can provide an accurate diagnosis and effective treatment for different types of depression.

1. Major Depressive Disorder

Major depressive disorder (MDD), also known as clinical depression, is a common and serious mood disorder that affects how a person feels, thinks, and behaves. It is characterized by persistent and pervasive feelings of sadness, hopelessness, and a loss of interest or pleasure in activities that were once enjoyable. These symptoms can interfere with daily activities, relationships, and work or school.

The symptoms of MDD can vary in severity and may include:

1. Feelings of sadness, emptiness, or hopelessness
2. Loss of interest or pleasure in activities once enjoyed
3. Significant weight loss or weight gain, or changes in appetite
4. Insomnia or excessive sleeping
5. Fatigue or loss of energy
6. Feelings of worthlessness or excessive guilt
7. Difficulty concentrating or making decisions
8. Recurrent thoughts of death or suicide

MDD can occur as a single episode or may be recurrent, with multiple episodes of depression separated by periods of normal mood. It can be caused by a combination of biological, environmental, and psychological factors, and may require treatment with medication, psychotherapy, or a combination of both.

It is important to seek professional help if experiencing symptoms of MDD, as early diagnosis and treatment can lead to better outcomes and improved quality of life.

2. Persistent Depressive Disorder

Persistent Depressive Disorder (PDD), also known as dysthymia, is a chronic type of depression that lasts for at least two years. It is characterized by a persistent feeling of sadness or low mood that is present most days and can interfere with daily activities.

The symptoms of PDD may include:

1. Feelings of sadness, hopelessness, or emptiness
2. Loss of interest or pleasure in activities once enjoyed
3. Low energy or fatigue

4. Changes in appetite or weight
5. Difficulty sleeping or oversleeping
6. Low self-esteem
7. Difficulty concentrating or making decisions
8. Feelings of hopelessness or pessimism

PDD is different from major depressive disorder (MDD) in that the symptoms are less severe but more chronic. It can be caused by a combination of biological, environmental, and psychological factors, and may require treatment with medication, psychotherapy, or a combination of both.

It is important to seek professional help if experiencing symptoms of PDD, as early diagnosis and treatment can lead to better outcomes and improved quality of life.

3. Bipolar Disorder

Bipolar disorder, also known as manic-depressive illness, is a mood disorder characterized by episodes of both depression and mania or hypomania. Bipolar disorder can affect a person's mood, energy, activity levels, and ability to function in daily life.

There are three main types of bipolar disorder:

1. Bipolar I Disorder: This type of bipolar disorder involves at least one manic episode, which is a period of abnormally elevated or irritable mood, lasting for at least one week. A person with bipolar I disorder may also experience depressive episodes.
2. Bipolar II Disorder: This type of bipolar disorder involves at least one episode of major depression and at least one hypomanic episode, which is a less severe form of mania that lasts for at least four days.
3. Cyclothymic Disorder: This type of bipolar disorder involves numerous periods of hypomanic symptoms and depressive symptoms lasting for at least two years in adults (one year in children and adolescents).

The symptoms of bipolar disorder can include:

1. Depressive symptoms: Feeling sad, hopeless, or empty, loss of interest in activities once enjoyed, changes in appetite and weight, difficulty

sleeping or oversleeping, low energy, feelings of worthlessness or guilt, difficulty concentrating or making decisions, and recurrent thoughts of death or suicide.

2. Manic symptoms: Feeling abnormally high or euphoric, increased energy and activity levels, racing thoughts, talking more than usual or talking quickly, inflated self-esteem or grandiosity, decreased need for sleep, impulsivity and poor judgement, and reckless or risky behavior.

Bipolar disorder is thought to be caused by a combination of genetic, biological, and environmental factors. It can be treated with medication, psychotherapy, or a combination of both, and with proper treatment, people with bipolar disorder can live healthy and productive lives.

4. Seasonal Affective Disorder

Seasonal Affective Disorder (SAD), also known as seasonal depression, is a type of depression that is related to changes in seasons, typically occurring in the fall and winter months. SAD is thought to be caused by the lack of sunlight during these months, which can disrupt the body's internal clock and affect the production of hormones like serotonin and melatonin.

The symptoms of SAD may include:

1. Feelings of sadness, hopelessness, or emptiness
2. Loss of interest or pleasure in activities once enjoyed
3. Low energy or fatigue
4. Changes in appetite or weight
5. Difficulty sleeping or oversleeping
6. Feelings of worthlessness or guilt
7. Difficulty concentrating or making decisions
8. Recurrent thoughts of death or suicide

SAD is often treated with light therapy, which involves exposure to a special light box that mimics outdoor light, and can help regulate the body's internal clock. Other treatments may include medication and psychotherapy.

It is important to seek professional help if experiencing symptoms of SAD, as early diagnosis and treatment can lead to better outcomes and improved quality of life.

XIII. Diagnosis of Depression

Diagnosis of depression usually involves a comprehensive assessment by a healthcare professional, such as a psychiatrist or psychologist. This assessment may include:

1. **Physical exam:** The healthcare professional may perform a physical exam to rule out any medical conditions that may be causing the symptoms.
2. **Psychological evaluation:** The healthcare professional may ask questions about the person's symptoms, thoughts, feelings, and behavior to determine if they meet the criteria for depression.
3. **Diagnostic criteria:** The healthcare professional may use criteria outlined in the Diagnostic and Statistical Manual of Mental Disorders (DSM-5) to diagnose depression. This includes the presence of certain symptoms for a specific length of time.
4. **Screening tools:** The healthcare professional may use screening tools, such as questionnaires or rating scales, to assess the severity of the symptoms and monitor progress over time.
5. **Family history:** The healthcare professional may ask about the person's family history of depression or other mental health conditions.

It is important to seek professional help if experiencing symptoms of depression, as early diagnosis and treatment can lead to better outcomes and improved quality of life.

1. Diagnostic criteria

The diagnostic criteria for depression as outlined in the Diagnostic and Statistical Manual of Mental Disorders (DSM-5) include the presence of one or both of the following:

1. **Depressed mood:** This can be expressed as feeling sad, empty, or hopeless, or losing interest or pleasure in most or all activities.
2. **Loss of interest or pleasure:** This can be expressed as a decreased interest in activities that were once enjoyable, or a decreased ability to feel pleasure from them.

In addition, the person must also have at least five of the following symptoms for a period of at least two weeks:

1. Significant weight loss or gain, or changes in appetite
2. Insomnia or hypersomnia
3. Psychomotor agitation or retardation
4. Fatigue or loss of energy
5. Feelings of worthlessness or excessive or inappropriate guilt
6. Diminished ability to think or concentrate, or indecisiveness
7. Recurrent thoughts of death or suicide, or a suicide attempt or plan

These symptoms must cause significant distress or impairment in social, occupational, or other areas of functioning.

It is important to note that the diagnosis of depression is based on the severity and duration of the symptoms, as well as the presence of functional impairment. A healthcare professional should be consulted for a comprehensive evaluation and diagnosis.

2. Assessment tools

There are several assessment tools that healthcare professionals may use to assess depression, including:

1. Beck Depression Inventory (BDI): This is a self-report questionnaire that assesses the severity of depressive symptoms. It includes 21 items that measure symptoms such as sadness, guilt, and loss of pleasure.
2. Patient Health Questionnaire (PHQ-9): This is a self-report questionnaire that assesses the severity of depressive symptoms over the past two weeks. It includes nine items that measure symptoms such as low mood, loss of interest, and sleep disturbances.
3. Hamilton Rating Scale for Depression (HAM-D): This is a clinician-administered rating scale that assesses the severity of depressive symptoms. It includes 21 items that measure symptoms such as depressed mood, insomnia, and suicidal ideation.
4. Geriatric Depression Scale (GDS): This is a self-report questionnaire that assesses depression in older adults. It includes 30 items that measure symptoms such as sadness, guilt, and social withdrawal.

5. Edinburgh Postnatal Depression Scale (EPDS): This is a self-report questionnaire that assesses depression in new mothers. It includes 10 items that measure symptoms such as low mood, anxiety, and suicidal ideation.

These assessment tools can help healthcare professionals to assess the severity of depressive symptoms and monitor progress over time. However, they should be used in conjunction with a comprehensive clinical evaluation and diagnosis by a healthcare professional.

XIV.Treatment for Depression

Depression is a treatable condition and there are several effective treatments available. The most common treatments for depression include:

1. Psychotherapy: Psychotherapy, also known as talk therapy, involves meeting with a mental health professional to discuss the thoughts, feelings, and behaviors that are contributing to depression. Different types of psychotherapy may be used, such as cognitive behavioral therapy (CBT), interpersonal therapy, or psychodynamic therapy.

2. Medication: Antidepressant medications, such as selective serotonin reuptake inhibitors (SSRIs) or serotonin-norepinephrine reuptake inhibitors (SNRIs), can be used to treat depression. These medications work by balancing the levels of neurotransmitters in the brain that are involved in mood regulation.

3. Electroconvulsive therapy (ECT): ECT is a treatment that involves applying brief electrical currents to the brain while the person is under anesthesia. This treatment is typically reserved for severe or treatment-resistant cases of depression.

4. Transcranial magnetic stimulation (TMS): TMS is a non-invasive treatment that uses magnetic fields to stimulate nerve cells in the brain. This treatment is typically used for people who have not responded to other treatments for depression.

5. Lifestyle changes: Making changes to lifestyle habits, such as getting regular exercise, eating a healthy diet, getting enough sleep, and reducing stress, can also help to alleviate symptoms of depression.

The most effective treatment for depression is often a combination of psychotherapy and medication. It is important to work with a healthcare professional to determine the best treatment plan for individual needs. In addition, self-help strategies, such as participating in social activities, practicing relaxation techniques, and setting achievable goals, can also be helpful in managing depression.

1. Medication

Medication is a common treatment option for depression. The most commonly prescribed medications for depression are antidepressants, such as selective serotonin reuptake inhibitors (SSRIs), serotonin-norepinephrine reuptake inhibitors (SNRIs), and tricyclic antidepressants (TCAs). These medications work by altering the levels of neurotransmitters in the brain, such as serotonin and norepinephrine, which are involved in regulating mood.

It is important to note that antidepressant medications can take several weeks to start working, and that not all medications work for everyone. It may be necessary to try several different medications, or a combination of medications, before finding an effective treatment.

In addition, it is important to work closely with a healthcare professional when taking antidepressant medication, as these medications can have side effects and may interact with other medications. Common side effects of antidepressant medications may include nausea, dry mouth, drowsiness, weight gain, or sexual dysfunction.

It is also important to note that medication should be used in conjunction with other treatments, such as psychotherapy, lifestyle changes, and self-help strategies, to achieve the best outcomes in managing depression.

2. Psychotherapy

Psychotherapy, also known as talk therapy, is a common treatment option for depression. It involves meeting with a mental health professional, such as a psychologist or therapist, to discuss thoughts, feelings, and behaviors that may be contributing to depression. There are several different types of psychotherapy that may be used to treat depression, including:

1. Cognitive behavioral therapy (CBT): CBT is a type of therapy that focuses on identifying negative thought patterns and behaviors that may be contributing to depression, and replacing them with more positive and adaptive ones.
2. Interpersonal therapy (IPT): IPT focuses on improving communication and relationship skills to help individuals with depression build better relationships and reduce social isolation.
3. Psychodynamic therapy: This type of therapy explores how past experiences and unresolved conflicts may be contributing to depression in the present.
4. Mindfulness-based cognitive therapy (MBCT): MBCT combines mindfulness techniques with cognitive therapy to help individuals with

depression learn to identify and change negative thought patterns.

5. Group therapy: Group therapy involves meeting with a group of individuals who are also experiencing depression and working together to support each other and learn coping skills.

Psychotherapy can be a highly effective treatment for depression, especially when used in combination with medication and other treatments. It is important to work with a trained mental health professional to determine the best type of therapy for individual needs and to ensure the best outcomes.

3. Lifestyle changes

Lifestyle changes can be an effective way to manage depression, and they may be used in conjunction with other treatments, such as medication and psychotherapy. Here are some lifestyle changes that may help manage depression:

1. Regular exercise: Exercise can help improve mood and reduce symptoms of depression. Even a small amount of exercise, such as a 30-minute walk, can be beneficial.
2. Healthy diet: Eating a balanced diet with plenty of fruits, vegetables, lean protein, and whole grains can help support overall health and reduce symptoms of depression.
3. Getting enough sleep: Sleep is essential for good mental health, and getting enough restful sleep can help improve mood and reduce symptoms of depression.
4. Stress management: Learning to manage stress through techniques such as mindfulness, meditation, or deep breathing exercises can help reduce symptoms of depression.
5. Social support: Having a strong support network of family and friends can help reduce feelings of isolation and loneliness, which are common in depression.
6. Avoiding alcohol and drugs: Alcohol and drug use can worsen symptoms of depression and interfere with the effectiveness of medications and other treatments.

It is important to work with a healthcare professional to develop a plan for lifestyle changes that are appropriate for individual needs and goals. While lifestyle changes alone may not be enough to manage severe depression, they can be a valuable tool in managing mild to moderate symptoms and promoting overall wellness.

4. Alternative treatments

There are several alternative treatments that may be used in conjunction with other treatments, such as medication and psychotherapy, to manage depression. Here are some alternative treatments that may be considered:

1. Acupuncture: Acupuncture involves inserting thin needles into specific points on the body to help alleviate symptoms of depression.
2. Herbal remedies: Certain herbal remedies, such as St. John's wort, may be used to treat mild to moderate depression. It is important to talk with a healthcare professional before taking any herbal remedies, as they can interact with other medications and may not be safe for everyone.
3. Yoga: Yoga combines physical postures, breathing techniques, and meditation to help reduce stress and improve mood.
4. Massage therapy: Massage therapy can help reduce stress and promote relaxation, which may help alleviate symptoms of depression.
5. Light therapy: Light therapy involves exposure to bright light to help alleviate symptoms of depression, especially seasonal affective disorder (SAD).

It is important to note that alternative treatments should be used in conjunction with, not as a replacement for, evidence-based treatments such as medication and psychotherapy. It is important to work with a healthcare professional to determine the best treatment plan for individual needs and goals.

<u>XV.Prevention of Depression</u>

Prevention of depression is an important consideration for individuals who may be at risk or have a history of depression. While there is no guaranteed way to prevent depression, there are some strategies that may be helpful:

1. Maintain a healthy lifestyle: Eating a healthy diet, exercising regularly, and getting enough restful sleep are all important for overall mental health and may help reduce the risk of developing depression.
2. Manage stress: Learning stress-management techniques, such as meditation, deep breathing exercises, or yoga, can help reduce stress and improve mood.
3. Build social support: Having a strong support network of family and friends can help reduce feelings of isolation and loneliness, which are risk factors for depression.
4. Identify and address early symptoms: It is important to be aware of early symptoms of depression, such as changes in sleep or appetite, feelings of sadness or hopelessness, or loss of interest in activities, and seek help as soon as possible.
5. Address underlying medical conditions: Certain medical conditions, such as thyroid disorders or chronic pain, can increase the risk of depression. It is important to work with a healthcare professional to manage any underlying medical conditions.
6. Consider therapy: Even individuals who have not been diagnosed with depression may benefit from therapy to help manage stress and improve overall mental health.

It is important to note that while these strategies may help reduce the risk of depression, they may not be effective for everyone. It is important to work with a healthcare professional to determine the best strategies for individual needs and goals.

1. Healthy lifestyle habits

Adopting healthy lifestyle habits is an important aspect of overall mental and physical health, and may help reduce the risk of depression. Here are some healthy lifestyle habits that may be helpful:

1. **Exercise regularly:** Exercise has been shown to improve mood and reduce symptoms of depression. Aim for at least 30 minutes of moderate-intensity exercise most days of the week.
2. **Eat a healthy diet**: Eating a balanced diet that includes plenty of fruits, vegetables, whole grains, lean protein, and healthy fats can provide essential nutrients for optimal mental and physical health.
3. **Get enough restful sleep:** Getting enough sleep is essential for overall health and wellbeing. Aim for 7-9 hours of restful sleep each night.
4. **Manage stress:** Learning stress-management techniques, such as meditation, deep breathing exercises, or yoga, can help reduce stress and improve mood.
5. **Build social support:** Having a strong support network of family and friends can help reduce feelings of isolation and loneliness, which are risk factors for depression.
6. **Limit alcohol and drug use:** Substance use can increase the risk of depression and other mental health problems. Limiting or avoiding alcohol and drug use can help improve overall mental health.
7. **Practice self-care:** Engaging in activities that promote relaxation and self-care, such as taking a warm bath, reading a book, or listening to music, can help reduce stress and improve mood.

It is important to note that while these healthy lifestyle habits may be helpful, they may not be effective for everyone. It is important to work with a healthcare professional to determine the best strategies for individual needs and goals.

• • • •

2. EARLY INTERVENTION and treatment

Early intervention and treatment is important for individuals with depression, as it can help improve symptoms and prevent the condition from worsening. Here are some reasons why early intervention and treatment is important:

1. <u>Reduced risk of complications:</u> Depression can lead to a number of complications, such as substance abuse, social isolation, and suicidal thoughts or behaviors. Early intervention and treatment can help reduce the risk of these complications.
2. **Improved outcomes:** Early treatment has been shown to improve outcomes for individuals with depression. Research suggests that early treatment can lead to a faster and more complete recovery, and may help prevent the condition from becoming chronic.
3. **Improved quality of life:** Depression can have a significant impact on an individual's quality of life, including their ability to function in daily activities and relationships. Early treatment can help improve mood, increase energy and motivation, and enhance overall quality of life.
4. **Reduced stigma:** Seeking treatment for depression can be challenging due to stigma and social attitudes towards mental illness. Early intervention and treatment can help reduce stigma and encourage individuals to seek help when they need it.
5. **Better overall health:** Depression can impact overall physical health, including immune function, cardiovascular health, and sleep quality. Early treatment can help improve overall health and prevent other health problems from developing.

It is important to seek help from a healthcare professional if you or a loved one is experiencing symptoms of depression. Early intervention and treatment can help improve outcomes and prevent the condition from worsening. Treatment may include medication, psychotherapy, lifestyle changes, and other supportive interventions.

XVI.Conclusion

Depression is a common mental health condition that can have a significant impact on an individual's life. It is important to understand the symptoms, causes, and types of depression in order to provide effective treatment and support. Seeking early intervention and treatment can help reduce the risk of complications and improve outcomes. Treatment may include medication, psychotherapy, lifestyle changes, and other supportive interventions. Adopting healthy lifestyle habits can also be helpful in reducing the risk of depression. It is important to work with a healthcare professional to determine the best strategies for individual needs and goals. With proper treatment and support, individuals with depression can lead healthy, fulfilling lives.

1. Summary of key points

Sure, here is a summary of the key points discussed in the outline:

- Depression is a mental health condition that can have emotional, physical, and behavioral symptoms.

- Biological, psychological, and environmental factors can contribute to depression.

- Major depressive disorder, persistent depressive disorder, bipolar disorder, and seasonal affective disorder are common types of depression.

- Diagnosis of depression may involve meeting certain criteria and the use of assessment tools.

- Treatment options for depression include medication, psychotherapy, lifestyle changes, and alternative treatments.

- Early intervention and treatment is important for reducing the risk of complications, improving outcomes, and enhancing quality of life.

- Healthy lifestyle habits and early intervention can help prevent depression.

- Seeking help from a healthcare professional is important for managing depression and developing an effective treatment plan.

2. Hope for recovery and future mental wellness for children and adolescents with depression

While depression can be a difficult and challenging experience for children and adolescents, it is important to remember that there is hope for recovery and future mental wellness. With proper diagnosis, treatment, and support, many children and adolescents with depression are able to overcome their symptoms and go on to live fulfilling and happy lives.

It is important to seek help and support from trained mental health professionals, as well as from family, friends, and support groups. Treatment options such as therapy, medication, and lifestyle changes can help alleviate symptoms and improve overall well-being. Encouraging open and honest communication, promoting healthy habits and activities, and being an advocate for your child or adolescent can also contribute to their recovery and long-term mental health.

While there may be challenges and controversies surrounding the treatment of depression in children and adolescents, it is important to remain hopeful and proactive in seeking the best care for your loved one. With a combination of professional support and personal dedication, there is potential for a brighter future for those struggling with depression.

3. Hope for individuals living with depression and anxiety

Living with depression and anxiety can be incredibly difficult, but it's important to remember that there is hope for recovery and a brighter future. While the journey to healing may not always be easy, there are effective treatments available and a supportive community of mental health professionals, loved ones, and peers who are ready to help. It's important to seek help early and to know that you are not alone in your struggles. With the right tools and support, it is possible to manage symptoms and achieve a fulfilling life. Remember, you are not defined by your mental health challenges, and there is always hope for a better tomorrow.

4. Encouragement to seek help for depression

If you or someone you know is experiencing symptoms of depression, it is important to seek help from a healthcare professional. Depression can be a serious condition that impacts every aspect of life, and it can be challenging to overcome without proper support and treatment.

Remember, seeking help is a sign of strength, not weakness. It takes courage to recognize when you need help and to take action towards improving your mental health. Healthcare professionals are trained to provide effective treatment and support, and can work with you to develop an individualized treatment plan.

Don't be afraid to reach out for help - there is no shame in seeking support for your mental health. With the right treatment and support, it is possible to manage depression and lead a fulfilling life. You deserve to feel happy, healthy, and fulfilled, and seeking help can be the first step towards achieving those goals.

Also by Swatantra Bahadur

1. Blossom with confidence
2. "Depression: A Roller Coaster Ride"
3. Finding Your Voice
4. Rahul Gandhi: The Untold Story
5. 100 Aspects on Nature
6. Love By An Introvert
7. Breaking Barriers: LGBTQ Rights and Social Justice
8. Man Of Golden India "Narendra Modi"
9. India " Unity lies in Diversity"
10. India's Heritage of Kashi "Varanasi"
11. "The Power of Voice: Lawyer in a Black Coat"
12. Shri Ram Janmabhumi "Ayodhya"
13. Social Media and Youth: Navigating the Digital Landscape
14. Jai Shri Hanuman Garhi "Ayodhya"
15. Chronicles of the Multiverse Cafe
16. "Unveiling Pain: The Global Impact of COVID-19

Website - Bookwisehub.com